CRANBERRY EXTRACT FOR BEGINNERS

Unlocking The Power Of Cranberry Extract, A Comprehensive Guide To Health Benefits, Usage, Wellness, Recipes, Vitality Enhancement And Beyond

Georgette Lockett

DISCLAIMER

The author of this book is not affiliated, associated, endorsed, sponsored, or approved by any company or individual. The views and opinions expressed in this book are solely those of the author and do not necessarily reflect the official policy or position of any entity.

The author hereby disclaims any relationship, collaboration, or partnership with any company or individual mentioned in this book. Any references to products, services, or individuals are provided for informational purposes only and should not be construed as an endorsement or recommendation.

Readers are advised to exercise their own judgment and discretion when applying the information provided in this book. The author shall not be held responsible for any actions taken by readers based on the content of this book.

This book is intended for general informational purposes only, and the author makes no representations or warranties of any kind, express or implied, about the completeness, accuracy, reliability, suitability, or availability of the information contained herein. Any reliance on the information in this book is at the reader's own risk.

The author reserves the right to update, change, or modify any information in this book without notice. It is the responsibility of the reader to verify any information before taking any actions based on the content of this book.

By reading this book, the reader acknowledges and agrees to the terms of this disclaimer.

Table of Contents

INTRODUCTION

Overview Of Cranberry Extract

The fruit of the cranberry plant (Vaccinium macrocarpon), a tiny, evergreen shrub native to North America, is used to make cranberry extract. Cranberries have long been appreciated for their brilliant red color, characteristic tart flavor, and remarkable list of health benefits. While cranberries are often ingested in a variety of forms such as fresh, dried, or juice, the extract provides a concentrated dosage of the fruit's beneficial ingredients.

Cranberry extract has a high concentration of phytochemicals, namely proanthocyanidins, which contribute to its antioxidant qualities. Because these components are thought to have several health advantages, cranberry extract has piqued the attention of both traditional medicine and scientific studies.

Importance And Uses

1. Urinary Tract Health: One of the key functions of cranberry extract is to promote urinary tract health. Certain chemicals in cranberries, according to research, may help reduce the adherence of bacteria, notably E. coli, to the urinary tract's walls. This anti-adhesive function may be especially useful in lowering the risk of urinary tract infections (UTIs), which are a frequent and recurring problem for many people.

2. Antioxidant Protection: Cranberry extract is high in antioxidants such as flavonoids and polyphenols. These chemicals are essential for neutralizing free radicals in the body and thereby lowering oxidative stress. Cranberry extract may contribute to overall cellular health and may have consequences for numerous chronic illnesses by decreasing the effect of oxidative stress.

3. Cardiovascular Support: According to a preliminary study, cranberry extract may offer cardiovascular advantages. Cranberries' antioxidants may help lower cholesterol and promote heart health. Furthermore, the anti-inflammatory effects of cranberry extract may help cardiovascular health.

4. Cranberry extract may have beneficial effects on gastrointestinal health in addition to its urinary and cardiovascular advantages. According to certain research, the anti-inflammatory and antioxidant characteristics of cranberry components may be beneficial in illnesses such as inflammatory bowel disease.

5. Dental Care: Cranberry extract's bioactive components may help with dental health. According to research, these substances may aid in inhibiting the adherence of certain bacteria to teeth, thereby lowering the incidence of dental plaque and cavities.

In conclusion, cranberry extract is a diverse natural substance that has a wide range of possible health advantages. Its uses range from urinary tract health promotion to cardiovascular function support and beyond. As we dive further into the complexities of cranberry extract, the next chapters will examine its mechanisms of action, clinical trials, and prospects in more depth, offering a thorough grasp of the potential that this modest berry has in the domain of health and wellness.

CHAPTER 1

Understanding Cranberries

Cranberry extract is a popular natural supplement made from the fruit of the cranberry plant, Vaccinium macrocarpon. Cranberries are native to North America and have been utilized for therapeutic purposes by Native American cultures long before European invaders arrived. They are known for their acidic flavor and brilliant red color. Cranberry extract has grown in popularity as a result of its possible health advantages and numerous uses.

History And Origins

Cranberries have been used for ages. Cranberries were used by Native American tribes such as the Wampanoag and Algonquin for a variety of reasons, including food, color, and medicinal. They preserved meat with cranberry paste, produced cranberry tea for its therapeutic properties, and utilized it as a natural color for garments and blankets.

Cranberries were famous in Europe in the 17th century, when they were known as "crane berries" due to the flower's resemblance to the head and beak of a crane. Cranberries, with their high vitamin C concentration, were frequently brought by sailors on their trips to avoid scurvy.

Botanical Information

Cranberries are low-growing shrubs of the Ericaceae family. These plants grow in colder, acidic, sandy bogs. They yield tiny, red berries in the autumn, which are collected. Cranberries have evergreen leaves and exquisite, bell-shaped pink blooms that emerge from late spring to early summer.

Nutritional Composition

Cranberries are well-known for their high nutritional content, which includes a variety of vitamins, minerals, and phytochemicals. They are high in vitamin C, vitamin A, and vitamin K. They also include dietary fibers like pectin and important minerals like manganese. Cranberries are also recognized for their strong antioxidant content, including flavonoids and phenolic compounds, which contribute to their potential health benefits.

Cranberries' active components, such as proanthocyanidins, are thought to promote urinary tract health by blocking the adherence of some bacteria to the urinary tract wall.

Cranberry extract is often concentrated to deliver increased quantities of beneficial chemicals generated from these nutrient-rich berries. To reap the potential health advantages of this extract, it is used in a variety of forms, including supplements, drinks, and powders.

Understanding the history, botanical features, and nutritional makeup of cranberries offers the groundwork for delving into the many applications and health advantages of cranberry extract.

CHAPTER 2

Health Benefits Of Cranberry Extract

Urinary Tract Health

Cranberry extract has received a lot of attention for its function in improving urinary tract health. It includes bioactive chemicals with anti-adhesive characteristics, such as proanthocyanidins (PACs). These chemicals inhibit the growth of some bacteria, mainly E. coli from sticking to the urinary system walls, lowering the incidence of urinary tract infections (UTIs). The anti-adhesive action prevents bacterial colonization in the bladder, which aids in the prevention and management of UTIs, particularly in women.

Antioxidant Properties

Cranberry Extract has significant antioxidant capabilities due to its high concentration of antioxidants such as flavonoids, polyphenols, and vitamins C and E. These chemicals scavenge free radicals in the body, reducing oxidative stress. Cranberry Extract may help general health by neutralizing damaging free radicals, thereby lowering the risk of chronic illnesses connected to oxidative stress, such as cancer, heart disease, and neurological ailments.

Potential Cardiovascular Benefits

According to research, the antioxidants in Cranberry Extract may benefit heart health. Regular ingestion may aid in the reduction of numerous cardiovascular risk factors. It may help decrease LDL cholesterol (the "bad" cholesterol), reduce inflammation, and improve blood vessel function.

These effects add up to a possibly decreased chance of acquiring cardiovascular illnesses.

Anti-Inflammatory Effects

Cranberry Extract has anti-inflammatory chemicals that may be useful in treating inflammatory diseases in the body. These anti-inflammatory properties may aid in the relief of symptoms associated with inflammatory disorders such as arthritis or gastrointestinal irritation.

Cranberry Extract is not only a tasty complement to a variety of cuisines and drinks, but it is also packed with health benefits. Its capacity to support urinary tract health by reducing bacterial adhesion, as well as its high antioxidant content, which combats oxidative stress, possible cardiovascular benefits, and anti-inflammatory qualities, all add to its importance in improving overall health and well-being.

As new information regarding Cranberry Extract's bioactive components and processes becomes available, it opens the door to new possible therapeutic uses. Cranberry Extract is a beneficial natural medicine because of its involvement in avoiding urinary tract infections, maintaining heart health, and reducing inflammation. Continued research and use of Cranberry Extract in different forms may give diverse health benefits, making it a crucial component in maintaining a healthy lifestyle.

CHAPTER 3

Cranberry Extract And Infections

Role In Preventing Urinary Tract Infections (Utis)

Cranberry extract has received a lot of attention for its ability to prevent and treat urinary tract infections (UTIs), owing to its bioactive components, notably proanthocyanidins (PACs) and other polyphenols. UTIs, which are often caused by the bacterium Escherichia coli (E. coli), are widespread, especially among women, and are linked with pain and frequent antibiotic use. Cranberry Extract is thought to inhibit E. coli adhesion. coli to the urinary tract wall, lowering the likelihood of infection. Bacterial colonization and subsequent infection are reduced by limiting bacterial adherence.

Several research have looked at the effectiveness of Cranberry Extract in preventing UTIs. However, the findings have been varied, with some studies indicating a possible benefit in certain groups (such as persistent UTI patients), while others show minimal efficacy. These results might be influenced by factors like as dose, active ingredient concentration, and the particular populations being investigated.

Other Bacterial Infections

Aside from UTIs, Cranberry Extract has shown potential in fighting a variety of bacterial diseases. Its anti-adhesive abilities may extend to other bacterial species, possibly inhibiting pathogen adhesion and colonization in other regions of the body, including the digestive system and mouth. This greater spectrum of action against bacterial adhesion might have consequences for gastrointestinal and oral infection prevention.

Supporting Scientific Evidence

The scientific data supporting Cranberry Extract's usefulness in preventing infections, particularly UTIs, is mixed. While some research supports its usage, others provide contradictory or equivocal outcomes. Variations in research design, Cranberry Extract formulations, doses, and participant demographics might explain the disparities in results.

A meta-analysis of clinical studies testing Cranberry Extract's effectiveness against UTIs, for example, revealed inconsistent findings. Some studies revealed a slight decrease in UTI incidence, particularly in select demographics, whereas others found no substantial effect. Variability in research methods, such as active component concentration, supplementation duration, and participant characteristics, may contribute to these disparities.

Despite discrepancies, Cranberry Extract's anti-adhesive effects remain an attractive field of study, with promise in preventing a variety of bacterial infections other than UTIs.

Understanding the mechanisms of action of Cranberry Extract and its influence on various bacterial strains and illness types is a topic of continuous research and clinical inquiry.

This chapter emphasizes the need to conduct more well-designed, large-scale clinical investigations to determine the specific function and efficiency of Cranberry Extract in preventing different bacterial illnesses. Furthermore, it emphasizes the significance of standardized formulations and doses in getting consistent outcomes and optimizing its therapeutic potential.

CHAPTER 4

Forms And Varieties Of Cranberry Extract

Juice Concentrate

Cranberry juice concentrate is a popular and widely accessible kind of cranberry extract. It is made by extracting cranberry juice and then evaporating the majority of the water content, resulting in a concentrated beverage. This form is popular due to its ease of use and adaptability. It is often used as a foundation for other drinks, such as cocktails and smoothies. Many of the beneficial elements present in whole cranberries, such as antioxidants and phytochemicals, are retained in the concentrate. However, because of the extraction procedure, it may be heavy in sugar and lack some nutrients found in whole cranberries.

Powder

Cranberry extract powder is made by drying and crushing cranberries into a fine powder. This form provides convenience and a longer shelf life. It's a frequent component in a variety of culinary applications, including baking, cooking, and even as a supplement. Cranberry powder may be combined into drinks, sprinkled over meals, or taken as a nutritional supplement in capsule form. It preserves many of the nutrients and bioactive chemicals found in fresh cranberries, making it an easy method to get the benefits of the fruit into one's diet.

Pills And Supplements

Cranberry extract is also available in pill, capsule, or tablet form, and is often advertised as a nutritional supplement. These supplements often include concentrated levels of cranberry extract, making it easier to consume the fruit's healthful ingredients in a more convenient and regulated manner.

Because of ingredients like proanthocyanidins, which may help inhibit bacterial adhesion in the urinary system, they are especially popular for their putative assistance in urinary tract health. The effectiveness of these supplements, however, may vary depending on the quality and quantity of active substances present.

Each kind of cranberry extract has its own set of benefits and drawbacks. Customers often choose the shape that best matches their interests and lifestyle. While juice concentrate makes for a delightful beverage, the powder gives flexibility in cooking and supplementing, and tablets or supplements provide convenience for focused health advantages. Understanding these different forms enables people to integrate cranberry extract into their daily routines based on their requirements and preferences.

CHAPTER 5

Dosage And Administration

Recommended Dosages

Because of its main ingredient, proanthocyanidins, which may prevent urinary tract infections (UTIs), cranberry extract is renowned for its possible health advantages. Cranberry Extract dose varies based on the formulation, concentration, and intended purpose of intake.

• For UTI prevention, it is customary for adults to take 500 mg to 1500 mg of Cranberry Extract in capsule or tablet form once or twice a day. This may differ depending on the severity of the UTI or different health circumstances.

• **For General Health Maintenance:** Lower dosages of Cranberry Extract, such as 300 mg to 400 mg per day, may be enough to promote urinary tract health while also delivering antioxidant benefits.

Ways To Consume Cranberry Extract

Cranberry Extract comes in a variety of forms, such as capsules, pills, powders, liquids, and dried extracts. The administration chosen is determined by personal preferences and the intended outcome:

• Cranberry Extract Capsules and Tablets: These are handy and give a regulated dose of Cranberry Extract. To guarantee effectiveness, make sure they contain a consistent quantity of the active components.

• Juices: Another approach to get the advantages is to drink pure, unsweetened cranberry juice. It is crucial to remember, however, that commercial cranberry drinks often have additional sugars, which may negate the health advantages.

• Powders and Dried Extracts: These may be used in smoothies, yogurt, or other dishes to suit personal tastes.

Precautions And Potential Side Effects

While moderate use of Cranberry Extract is usually regarded as safe for most individuals, there are a few things to bear in mind:

• **Allergies:** People who are sensitive to aspirin may have a similar response to cranberries owing to the presence of salicylic acid. In such instances, it is best to avoid cranberry products.

• **Blood Thinners:** Cranberry may interact with blood thinners such as warfarin, thereby raising the risk of bleeding. If you are using such drugs, you should consult with a healthcare provider before beginning Cranberry Extract.

• **Stomach upset:** High dosages of Cranberry Extract may induce stomach pain or diarrhea in some people. To measure tolerance, it is advisable to begin with smaller dosages and progressively increases.

- **Interaction with Kidney Stones:** Oxalates in cranberry extract may lead to the production of kidney stones in sensitive people. Those with a history of kidney stones should reduce their intake.

Before beginning any new supplement regimen, visit a healthcare practitioner, particularly if you have underlying health concerns or are taking drugs, to avoid possible interactions and ensure an adequate dose.

Understanding the appropriate doses, modes of ingestion, and precautions is critical for the safe and efficient use of Cranberry Extract to optimize its potential health benefits while reducing hazards.

CHAPTER 6

Cranberry Extract In Culinary And Home Remedies

Recipes Incorporating Cranberry Extract

1. **Cranberry Sauce:** Cranberry sauce mixes the acidity of cranberries with sugar or sweeteners to provide a tasty complement to roast turkey, poultry, or even as a spread in sandwiches.

2. **Cranberry Smoothie:** Combine cranberry extract with fruits such as strawberries and bananas, as well as a splash of yogurt or almond milk, to make a healthy and tart smoothie high in antioxidants and vitamins.

3. **Cranberry-Orange Bread:** For a delectable dessert or brunch treat, combine dried cranberries or cranberry essence with moist, citrusy bread.

4. Cranberry-Glazed fish: Make a sweet and savory glaze with cranberry extract, honey, and a splash of soy sauce for baked or grilled fish.

5. Cranberry Salad Dressing: Combine cranberry extract, olive oil, balsamic vinegar, Dijon mustard, and herbs to make a spicy salad dressing.

DIY Home Remedies

1. Tonic for Urinary Tract Health: Cranberry extract is well-known for its ability to improve urinary tract health. Make your tonic by combining cranberry extract with water or apple juice. By preventing germs from sticking to the bladder walls, it may help to avoid urinary tract infections.

2. Antioxidant Face Mask: To make a revitalizing face mask, combine cranberry extract, honey, and plain yogurt. Cranberries are high in antioxidants, which may aid in brightening skin and minimize the appearance of blemishes.

3. Make a homemade hair rinse using cranberry extract to give luster and manageability to your strands. After shampooing, combine cranberry extract and water for a refreshing rinse.

4. Cranberry Infusion for Digestive Health: Make a calming tea with cranberry extract and additional herbs like ginger or mint for digestion and gut health.

The adaptability of cranberry extract goes beyond conventional recipes, providing a variety of creative options for both culinary pleasures and holistic home treatments. Its rich flavor and possible health advantages make it an excellent complement to a variety of handmade dishes, satisfying both taste buds and well-being.

CHAPTER 7

Research And Studies

Overview Of Scientific Research

Cranberry extract has piqued the curiosity of scientists due to its possible health advantages. Researchers have studied its features to better understand its methods of action, effectiveness, and potential uses in a variety of health disorders. Its chemical contents have been studied, with an emphasis on the active molecules responsible for its health-promoting benefits, including proanthocyanidins, flavonoids, and organic acids.

Clinical Trials And Findings

Numerous clinical studies have been conducted to explore the effectiveness of cranberry extract in a variety of health areas:

1. **Urinary Tract Health:** Urinary tract health is perhaps the most well-known topic of inquiry. Cranberry extract has been widely researched for its ability to reduce urinary tract infections (UTIs). Findings have been mixed, however, some studies show that cranberry components may interfere with bacterium adherence to the urinary system, lowering the likelihood of infection.

2. Cranberry extract, which is high in antioxidants, has been researched for its ability to counteract oxidative stress. Its polyphenol content, particularly proanthocyanidins, has high antioxidant activity, which may contribute to a variety of health advantages such as cardiovascular health and anti-inflammatory properties.

3. Emerging research suggests that the bioactive components found in cranberry extract may be beneficial to gastrointestinal health. Its significance in modifying gut flora, lowering the incidence of

stomach ulcers, and increasing digestive health is being studied.

4. Dental Health: Some research suggests that cranberry extract may limit oral bacteria attachment to teeth, thereby lowering the risk of dental plaque buildup and gum disease.

5. Cardiovascular Health: Cranberry extract polyphenols have attracted attention to their possible cardiovascular advantages, including improving lipid profiles and lowering the risk of atherosclerosis.

Ongoing Studies And Future Prospects

The topic of cranberry extract research is still evolving, with current studies investigating numerous aspects:

1. Precision Medicine: Researchers are investigating tailored methods for cranberry extract use, taking into account characteristics such as individual genetic makeup and gut microbiota composition to maximize its advantages for certain groups.

2. Novel Applications: Ongoing research attempts to identify new potential applications for cranberry extract beyond its current usage. This involves investigating its possible involvement in immunological support, cognitive health, and anti-cancer capabilities.

3. Standardization and Quality Control: Efforts are underway to standardize cranberry extract formulations to ensure consistent quality and potency for research and commercial goods.

4. Combination Therapies: Researchers are looking at possible synergies between cranberry extract and other natural components or medicines to improve therapeutic effects.

To summarize, although cranberry extract shows promise in a variety of health areas, more well-designed clinical trials and rigorous research are required to completely unravel its mechanisms of action, improve dose regimens, and broaden its uses in preventive and therapeutic medicine. The continuous investigation of cranberry extract's potential across numerous health fronts emphasizes its importance as a topic of ongoing scientific investigation and prospective health assistance.

CHAPTER 8

Choosing The Right Cranberry Extract

Cranberry extract has gained popularity owing to its possible health advantages, notably in the support of urinary tract health and the prevention of infections. However, choosing the most efficient and dependable cranberry extract may be difficult owing to market variances in quality, strength, and sources.

Quality Considerations

1. **Purity:** Make certain that the cranberry extract is devoid of impurities, additions, or fillers that might reduce its efficacy. Look for items that have been thoroughly purified.

2. Select extracts that have been standardized to have high amounts of active chemicals, such as proanthocyanidins (PACs).

The molecules known as PACs are thought to add to the health advantages of cranberries.

3. Consider extracts prepared from high-quality cranberry fruits grown in clean conditions free of pesticides and toxins. Cold pressing or gentle solvent extraction procedures generally maintain bioactive components better than severe treatments.

4. **Third-party Testing:** Look for items that have been independently tested for potency, purity, and safety by a third party. Certifications or seals from organizations like NSF, USP, or ConsumerLab may indicate the quality of a product.

Label Information To Look For

1. **PAC Content:** Check the label for the quantity of proanthocyanidins. A trustworthy product should disclose the PAC concentration, which is commonly measured in milligrams per serving.

2. Components: Make sure the extract includes just pure cranberry and no other components. Avoid extracts that include superfluous additions or preservatives.

3. Production Specifications: Look for details on the production process, extraction technique, and any quality certifications or testing that have been performed.

Finding Reliable Sources

1. Repute and Reviews: Look into the brand's or manufacturer's repute. User reviews, expert recommendations, and testimonials may provide information about the product's quality and effectiveness.

2. Consult Experts: Seek counsel from healthcare specialists or herbal supplement experts. They may advise you on recognized brands or specialized compositions depending on your requirements.

3. Companies that give openness about their sourcing, production procedures, and quality control systems are more likely to supply trustworthy goods.

Finally, choosing a high-quality cranberry extract requires careful evaluation of purity, standardization, label information, and the source's reliability. A well-informed decision may have a considerable influence on the extract's efficacy in offering possible cranberry health advantages. Before beginning any new supplement regimen, always speak with a healthcare expert.

CHAPTER 9

Cranberry Extract And General Wellness

Supplementary Benefits

1. Urinary Tract Health: Cranberry extract is well-known for its potential to improve urinary tract health. Cranberries' high proanthocyanidin (PAC) concentration inhibits the adhesion of some bacteria, notably E. coli. coli to the urinary tract walls, lowering the incidence of UTIs. Regular use or supplementation with cranberry extract may help to alleviate or prevent UTIs.

2. Antioxidant Properties: Cranberries have a high concentration of antioxidants such as flavonoids, polyphenols, and vitamins C and E. These antioxidants protect the organism from oxidative stress by neutralizing free radicals. This characteristic may aid in the reduction of cell damage, the maintenance of immunological function, and the prevention of chronic illnesses.

3. **Cardiovascular Health:** Cranberry extract's antioxidants may benefit cardiovascular health by possibly lowering risk factors for heart disease. They may help reduce blood pressure, improve cholesterol levels, and promote general heart health.

4. **Digestive Health:** Cranberry compounds such as flavonoids and dietary fiber may benefit gastrointestinal health. They may support good digestion, relieve gastrointestinal pain, and maybe contribute to a balanced gut microbiota.

Integrating Into A Healthy Lifestyle

Incorporating cranberry extract into one's regimen may be part of a comprehensive approach to overall well-being. Some strategies to include it in a healthy lifestyle are as follows:

• **Supplementation:** For people looking for specific health advantages, using cranberry extract as a supplement may provide standardized quantities of beneficial components.

• **Dietary Inclusion:** Including whole cranberries or cranberry-derived products in one's diet may provide nutritional and antioxidant advantages. This may be accomplished by the use of liquids, dried cranberries, or the incorporation of fresh cranberries into meals.

• **Hydration:** Cranberry juice, a popular option, maybe a healthy alternative to sugary drinks, increasing hydration while also offering antioxidants.

Potential Synergies With Other Supplements

Cranberry extract may be used in conjunction with other supplements or dietary ingredients to improve overall health:

• Probiotics: Combining cranberry extract with probiotics may benefit gut health by establishing a healthy microbiota and assisting with digestion.

• Vitamin C: Cranberry extract and vitamin C supplements may work together to promote immune function and provide greater antioxidant protection.

• Omega-3 Fatty Acids: Cranberry extract, when used with omega-3 supplements, may help to cardiovascular health by possibly decreasing inflammation and lowering the risk of heart disease.

CHAPTER 10

Consumer Guide And Frequently Asked Questions (Faqs)

Buying Guide

When buying cranberry extract, keep the following criteria in mind to guarantee quality and effectiveness:

1. Select extracts that have been standardized for active chemicals such as proanthocyanidins (PACs). Look for supplements that have few fillers or chemicals.

2. Formulation: Choose the appropriate form for you: capsules, pills, liquid extracts, or powders.

3. Ingredients: Look for items with a low amount of added sugar or artificial additives. Organic alternatives may also be offered.

4. Choose items from reputable producers with a proven track record of quality and safety.

Commonly Asked Questions And Answers

Q: What active ingredients are in cranberry extract? A: Cranberry extract includes bioactive components called proanthocyanidins (PACs), which are thought to benefit urinary tract health by preventing bacterial attachment to the bladder wall.

Q: What are the possible health advantages of cranberry extract? A: Cranberry extract is well-known for its ability to improve urinary tract health by lowering the risk of urinary tract infections (UTIs). It also has antioxidant capabilities, which may be beneficial to general health.

Q: How should I drink cranberry extract? A: The suggested dose varies depending on the product and the person. Follow the directions on the product label or get advice from a healthcare expert.

Can cranberry extract help to prevent UTIs? A: Cranberry extract includes chemicals that may prevent some germs from adhering to the urinary system walls, thereby lowering the incidence of UTIs. It is not, however, a guaranteed preventative strategy and should not be used instead of approved therapies.

Q: Does cranberry extract have any negative side effects? A: When consumed in suitable proportions, cranberry extract is generally safe for most individuals. Excessive consumption, on the other hand, may cause stomach distress or diarrhea in certain people. Because cranberry extract has the potential to alter blood clotting, those on blood-thinning drugs should see a healthcare practitioner before taking it.

Tips For Maximum Benefits

1. **Maintain Adequate Water consumption:** Adequate water consumption supplements the benefits of cranberry extract in promoting urinary health.

2. Maintaining a regular intake pattern may be advantageous for people utilizing cranberry extract to enhance urinary health.

3. **Visit a Professional:** Before beginning any new supplement, always visit a healthcare practitioner, particularly if you have pre-existing medical issues or are using drugs.

Finally, cranberry extract has grown in popularity as a result of its possible advantages for urinary tract health and general well-being. When selecting a supplement, choose high-quality goods, adhere to stated amounts, and seek expert counsel for individualized guidance. Cranberry extract may be a helpful complement to a health-conscious lifestyle when used and cared for properly.

Conclusion

Cranberry extract, a product extracted from the brilliant red cranberry fruit, has piqued the interest of consumers owing to its many advantages and medical capabilities.

Recap Of Key Points

Several critical characteristics of cranberry extract have surfaced throughout this investigation. Cranberries, which originated in North America, have a long history of usage by indigenous peoples for their healing effects. Cranberries, a member of the Vaccinium genus, have a botanical history that highlights their distinctive traits and development patterns in acidic, bog-like settings.

Cranberries have an interesting nutritional profile. These fruits are high in antioxidants, namely flavonoids and polyphenols, which are known for their potential health advantages.

Cranberry extract is also high in vitamins C, A, and K, as well as minerals like manganese and fiber, which adds to its nutritious value.

Cranberry extract has a wide range of health advantages. One of its most well-known uses is supporting urinary tract health by possibly avoiding urinary tract infections (UTIs) via anti-adhesive qualities against specific bacteria. Furthermore, its antioxidant capabilities have piqued the curiosity of researchers interested in its possible function in cardiovascular health, cancer prevention, and dental health. Studies also indicate that it has anti-inflammatory and gastrointestinal health benefits.

Aside from its health benefits, cranberry extract's versatility finds use in the food and beverage sector, cosmetics, and medicines, emphasizing its economic value.

The future of cranberry extract seems bright as the study continues. More research into its mechanisms of action, absorption, and appropriate dose will help to optimize its medicinal uses. Understanding its potential in treating rising health issues and investigating novel applications beyond its usual usage is an intriguing field for academics to explore.

Furthermore, innovations in extraction processes and formulations may increase the potency and effectiveness of cranberry extract, opening up new avenues for its incorporation into many healthcare sectors.

Finally, cranberry extract is a monument to the tremendous combination of nature's wealth and medical potential. Its wide range of health advantages, along with its commercial adaptability, highlight its importance in contemporary health and industry. Continued study and use of cranberry extract is critical to realize its full potential and pave the way for a healthier future.

THE END